LOW FAT

FOOD LIST

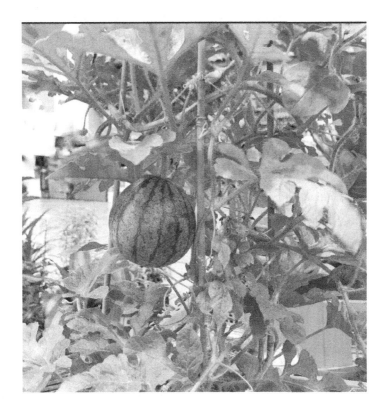

LORENE PEACHEY

DISCLAIMER

The content within this book reflects my thoughts, experiences, and beliefs. It is meant for informational and entertainment purposes. While I have taken great care to provide accurate information, I cannot guarantee the absolute correctness or applicability of the content to every individual or situation. Please consult with relevant professionals for advice specific to your needs.

TO GAIN ACCESS TO MORE BOOK BY THE AUTHOR SCAN THE QR CODE

TABLE OF CONTENTS

INTRODUCTION

In the quiet corners of my kitchen, where flavors dance and ingredients fuse into culinary symphonies, my journey as a nutritionist, Lorene Peachey, has unfolded over the span of a quarter-century. I am not just a connoisseur of food; I am an artist sculpting a masterpiece that celebrates health and vitality. Welcome to my world, where Low Fat isn't just a dietary choice; it's a way of life, a devotion that has transformed my existence into a canvas painted with the vibrant hues of well-being.

For as long as I can remember, I have been fascinated by the power of food—its ability to heal, nourish, and uplift. My odyssey into the realm of nutritional recipes began with a simple question: Can food be a source of not just pleasure but profound well-being? Armed with curiosity and a passion for wholesome living, I embarked on a quest to uncover the secrets of crafting recipes that not only tantalize the taste buds but also nurture the body and soul.

Picture this: a kitchen filled with the aromas of fresh herbs, the sizzle of vibrant vegetables, and the promise of a meal that transcends mere sustenance. It was within these walls that I delved into the world of Low Fat, a culinary philosophy that would become my life's work. As a nutritionist, my mission became clear—to create a repertoire of recipes that marry deliciousness with healthfulness, where each bite isn't just a burst of flavor but a step towards a vibrant and energized life.

Over the years, I have poured my heart and soul into deciphering the intricacies of nutritional science, dissecting the benefits of low-fat living. It wasn't merely a profession; it became a calling, a responsibility to guide others on the path to wholesome living. With each recipe crafted, I found fulfillment in knowing that I wasn't just offering a meal but a roadmap to a healthier, more vibrant existence.

But why Low Fat? Why the relentless pursuit of recipes that trim away the unnecessary and elevate the essential? The answers to these questions lie in the emotional core of our well-being. Consider this: have you ever felt the invigorating surge of energy that accompanies a meal rich in nutrients and devoid of excessive fats? Have you experienced the joy of savoring a dish that not only satiates your taste buds but leaves you feeling light and revitalized?

These are not mere sensations; they are the emotional echoes of a body nourished, a spirit lifted. In the tapestry of our lives, food weaves its threads intricately, influencing not just our physical health but our emotional well-being. The questions I pose aren't just rhetorical; they are an invitation to reflect on the profound connection between what we eat and how we feel.

Now, let's confront a harsh truth—one that often hides behind the allure of decadent indulgence. What are the consequences of feasting on a diet laden with unhealthy fats, sugars, and processed foods? Picture the heaviness that settles in your gut, the sluggishness that clouds your mind, and the guilt that lingers like a shadow. It's a reality many face—a consequence of the modern lifestyle, the hurried pace that often sacrifices health at the altar of convenience.

This brings us to the heart of the matter—the benefits of embracing a Low-Fat food list. Beyond the obvious advantages of weight management and cardiovascular health, consider the emotional dividends. Imagine waking up with a lightness of being, free from the burdens of a body weighed down by excess. Envision the clarity that accompanies a well-nourished mind, the vigor that propels you through the day, and the confidence that radiates from a body in harmony.

In my culinary laboratory, I've seen the transformational power of Low-Fat recipes. The joyous testimonials from individuals who embarked on this journey speak louder than any scientific study. It's about more than just numbers on a scale; it's about reclaiming your vitality, rediscovering the pleasure in nourishing your body, and experiencing the boundless energy that arises from wholesome living.

Allow me to share a revelation that stems from two and a half decades of unwavering dedication—Low Fat living isn't a sacrifice; it's a liberation. It liberates you from the shackles of unhealthy choices, from the tyranny of excess, and from the limitations that a tired, lethargic body imposes. It is an act of self-love, a daily affirmation that you deserve the very best life has to offer.

Now, let's talk about my Low-Fat food list—a treasure trove of culinary delights that redefine the concept of dieting. Picture a plate adorned with Grilled Lemon Herb Chicken, its succulence enhanced by a marinade that whispers of citrusy zest and fragrant herbs. Visualize the vibrancy of a Quinoa and Black Bean Salad, a melody of colors and textures that dances on your palate.

But it's not just about the dishes; it's about the symphony of nutrients they bring to your body. Imagine the antioxidants in every bite, the fiber that nourishes your digestive system, and the proteins that build and repair. It's not just a meal; it's a nutritional symphony that harmonizes with your body's needs, a feast that transcends the mundane and embraces the extraordinary.

In this gastronomic odyssey, you'll encounter the exquisite notes of Baked Lemon Garlic Tilapia, the comforting warmth of Lentil and Vegetable Soup, and the invigorating crunch of Shrimp and Vegetable Stir-Fry. These aren't just recipes; they are invitations to a culinary adventure that promises not just satiation but a celebration of life.

My journey, intertwined with yours through the pages of this book, is a testament to the enduring power of food as medicine. It's a journey of self-discovery, an exploration of the profound link between what we consume and how we feel. As you embark on this 21-day odyssey of Low-Fat living, consider it not just a dietary shift but a holistic transformation—a commitment to nurturing not just your body but your soul.

So, dear reader, are you ready to savor the delights of Low-Fat living? Are you prepared to bid farewell to the heaviness that comes with unhealthy choices and embrace the buoyancy that accompanies wholesome living? As you delve into the chapters that unfold before you, let the aromas wafting from the pages tantalize your senses, and the words resonate as a friendly guide on your journey to vitality.

And remember this—every recipe, every morsel, is a step towards a brighter, healthier tomorrow. Let the culinary adventure begin!

Contact the Author

Thank you for reading my book! I would love to hear from you, whether you have feedback, questions, or just want to share your thoughts. Your feedback means a lot to me and helps me improve as a writer.

Please don't hesitate to reach out to me through

lorenepeachey@gmail.com

I look forward to connecting with my readers and appreciate your support in this literary journey. Your thoughts and comments are valuable to me.

CHAPTER 1

OVERVIEW OF LOW-FAT DIET

A low-fat diet is a nutritional approach that focuses on reducing the intake of dietary fats, especially saturated and trans fats. The primary goal of this diet is to promote overall health by lowering the risk of certain chronic conditions such as heart disease, obesity, and high cholesterol levels. In a low-fat diet, individuals aim to replace high-fat foods with nutrient-rich alternatives, emphasizing a balance of carbohydrates, proteins, and healthy fats.

Benefits of a Low-Fat Lifestyle:

1. **Heart Health:** Reduced consumption of saturated and trans fats can contribute to lower levels of LDL cholesterol, often referred to as "bad" cholesterol. This, in turn, supports cardiovascular health and lowers the risk of heart disease.

2. **Weight Management:** A low-fat diet can be effective for weight control, as it typically involves a lower calorie intake. By choosing foods that are lower in fat, individuals can create a calorie deficit, helping to manage or lose weight when combined with regular physical activity.

3. **Improved Blood Sugar Control:** For individuals with or at risk of diabetes, a low-fat diet may help regulate blood sugar levels. Choosing complex carbohydrates and lean proteins over high-fat options can contribute to better insulin sensitivity.

4. **Cancer Prevention:** Some studies suggest that a low-fat diet may be associated with a reduced risk of certain types of cancer, including breast and colon cancer. However, more research is needed to establish conclusive evidence.

5. **Digestive Health:** A diet rich in fruits, vegetables, and whole grains, which are often part of a low-fat lifestyle, can promote digestive health by providing essential fiber and nutrients.

6. **Long-Term Health:** Adopting a low-fat lifestyle may contribute to long-term health and well-being, reducing the likelihood of developing chronic diseases associated with high-fat diets.

CHAPTER 2

UNDERSTANDING FATS

Understanding Fats

Fats are essential components of a balanced diet, playing crucial roles in maintaining overall health and well-being. They are a type of macronutrient, along with carbohydrates and proteins. Fats are concentrated sources of energy, providing more than twice the calories per gram compared to carbohydrates and proteins. It is important to understand the different types of dietary fats, their functions in the body, and the recommended daily fat intake for optimal health.

Types of Dietary Fats:

1. **Saturated Fats:**

    - Found in animal products such as meat, dairy, and certain tropical oils.

    - Consuming excessive saturated fats may contribute to an increase in LDL cholesterol levels, potentially raising the risk of heart disease.

2. **Unsaturated Fats:**

- Monounsaturated Fats: Present in olive oil, avocados, and certain nuts.

- Polyunsaturated Fats: Found in fatty fish, walnuts, flaxseeds, and vegetable oils.

- Both types of unsaturated fats can have positive effects on heart health when consumed in moderation.

3. **Trans Fats:**

- Artificially created through hydrogenation, often found in processed and fried foods.

- Trans fats can raise LDL cholesterol and lower HDL cholesterol, increasing the risk of heart disease. Many health organizations recommend minimizing their consumption.

The Role of Fats in the Body:

1. **Energy Source:**

   - Fats serve as a concentrated source of energy, particularly during periods of low food intake or intense physical activity.

2. **Cell Structure:**

   - Fats are crucial components of cell membranes, contributing to their structure and function.

3. **Nutrient Absorption:**

   - Certain vitamins (A, D, E, and K) are fat-soluble, meaning they require fats for absorption. Fats facilitate the absorption of these vitamins in the digestive system.

4. **Insulation and Protection:**

   - Adipose tissue, which stores fat, acts as insulation and protects vital organs in the body.

5. **Hormone Production:**

   - Fats are involved in the production of hormones, including sex hormones and hormones that regulate metabolism.

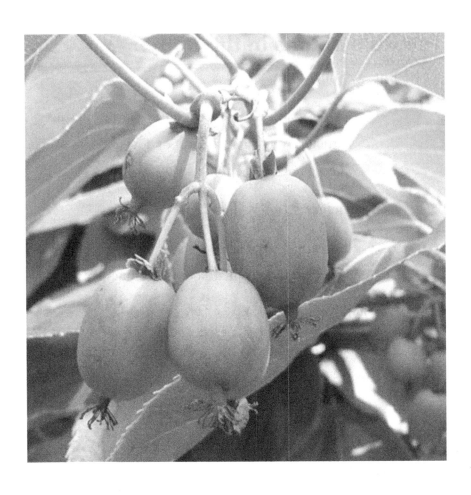

CHAPTER 3

LOW-FAT PROTEINS

1. **Chicken Breast:**

   - Nutritional Information (per 3.5 ounces):

     - Calories: 165

     - Protein: 31g

     - Total Fat: 3.6g

     - Saturated Fat: 1g

2. **Turkey Breast:**

   - Nutritional Information (per 3.5 ounces):

     - Calories: 135

     - Protein: 30g

     - Total Fat: 1g

     - Saturated Fat: 0.3g

3. **Fish (Cod or Haddock):**

- Nutritional Information (per 3.5 ounces):

    - Calories: 95

    - Protein: 20g

    - Total Fat: 1g

    - Saturated Fat: 0.2g

4. **Greek Yogurt (Non-fat):**

- Nutritional Information (per 1 cup):

    - Calories: 100

    - Protein: 22g

    - Total Fat: 0g

    - Saturated Fat: 0g

5. **Cottage Cheese (Low-fat):**

- Nutritional Information (per 1 cup):

    - Calories: 210

    - Protein: 28g

    - Total Fat: 4g

    - Saturated Fat: 2.5g

6. **Egg Whites:**

- Nutritional Information (per 3.5 ounces):

    - Calories: 52

    - Protein: 11g

    - Total Fat: 0g

    - Saturated Fat: 0g

7. **Beans (Black Beans, Kidney Beans):**

- Nutritional Information (per 1 cup, cooked):

    - Calories: 220

    - Protein: 15g

    - Total Fat: 1g

    - Saturated Fat: 0g

8. **Lentils:**

- Nutritional Information (per 1 cup, cooked):

    - Calories: 230

    - Protein: 18g

    - Total Fat: 0.8g

    - Saturated Fat: 0.1g

9. **Tofu:**

- Nutritional Information (per 3.5 ounces):

    - Calories: 144

    - Protein: 15g

    - Total Fat: 8g

    - Saturated Fat: 1.1g

10. **Skinless Turkey or Chicken Drumsticks:**

- Nutritional Information (per 3.5 ounces):

    - Calories: 135

    - Protein: 28g

    - Total Fat: 3.5g

    - Saturated Fat: 1g

CHAPTER 4

HEALTHY CARBOHYDRATES

1. **Sweet Potatoes:**

   - Nutritional Information (per 1 cup, mashed):

     - Calories: 180

     - Carbohydrates: 41g

     - Dietary Fiber: 6g

     - Total Fat: 0.3g

     - Saturated Fat: 0.1g

2. **Quinoa:**

   - Nutritional Information (per 1 cup, cooked):

     - Calories: 222

     - Carbohydrates: 39g

     - Dietary Fiber: 5g

     - Total Fat: 4g

     - Saturated Fat: 0.4g

3. **Oats:**

  - Nutritional Information (per 1 cup, cooked):

    - Calories: 147

    - Carbohydrates: 25g

    - Dietary Fiber: 4g

    - Total Fat: 2.5g

    - Saturated Fat: 0.5g

4. **Brown Rice:**

  - Nutritional Information (per 1 cup, cooked):

    - Calories: 218

    - Carbohydrates: 45g

    - Dietary Fiber: 4g

    - Total Fat: 1.6g

    - Saturated Fat: 0.3g

5. **Quinoa:**

- Nutritional Information (per 1 cup, cooked):

    - Calories: 222

    - Carbohydrates: 39g

    - Dietary Fiber: 5g

    - Total Fat: 4g

    - Saturated Fat: 0.4g

6. **Lentils:**

- Nutritional Information (per 1 cup, cooked):

    - Calories: 230

    - Carbohydrates: 40g

    - Dietary Fiber: 16g

    - Total Fat: 1g

    - Saturated Fat: 0.1g

7. **Chickpeas:**

- Nutritional Information (per 1 cup, cooked):

    - Calories: 269

    - Carbohydrates: 45g

    - Dietary Fiber: 12g

    - Total Fat: 4g

    - Saturated Fat: 0.4g

8. **Barley:**

- Nutritional Information (per 1 cup, cooked):

    - Calories: 193

    - Carbohydrates: 44g

    - Dietary Fiber: 6g

    - Total Fat: 1g

    - Saturated Fat: 0.1g

9. **Whole Wheat Pasta:**

- Nutritional Information (per 1 cup, cooked):

  - Calories: 174

  - Carbohydrates: 37g

  - Dietary Fiber: 6g

  - Total Fat: 1g

  - Saturated Fat: 0.1g

10. **Black Beans:**

- Nutritional Information (per 1 cup, cooked):

  - Calories: 227

  - Carbohydrates: 41g

  - Dietary Fiber: 15g

  - Total Fat: 0.9g

  - Saturated Fat: 0.2g

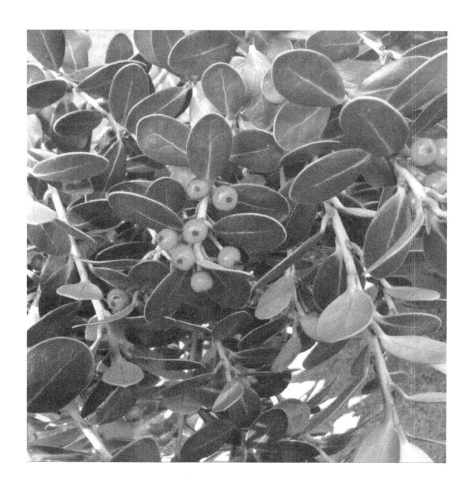

CHAPTER 5

FRUITS

1. **Strawberries:**

    - Nutritional Information (per cup, sliced):

        - Calories: 50

        - Carbohydrates: 12g

        - Dietary Fiber: 3g

        - Total Fat: 0.5g

        - Saturated Fat: 0g

2. **Watermelon:**

    - Nutritional Information (per cup, diced):

        - Calories: 46

        - Carbohydrates: 12g

        - Dietary Fiber: 0.6g

        - Total Fat: 0.2g

        - Saturated Fat: 0g

3. **Papaya:**

- Nutritional Information (per cup, diced):

    - Calories: 59

    - Carbohydrates: 15g

    - Dietary Fiber: 3g

    - Total Fat: 0.4g

    - Saturated Fat: 0.1g

4. **Cantaloupe:**

- Nutritional Information (per cup, diced):

    - Calories: 54

    - Carbohydrates: 14g

    - Dietary Fiber: 1.6g

    - Total Fat: 0.3g

    - Saturated Fat: 0g

5. **Grapefruit:**

- Nutritional Information (per half, medium-sized):

    - Calories: 52

    - Carbohydrates: 13g

    - Dietary Fiber: 2g

    - Total Fat: 0.2g

    - Saturated Fat: 0g

6. **Kiwi:**

- Nutritional Information (per medium-sized):

    - Calories: 61

    - Carbohydrates: 15g

    - Dietary Fiber: 3g

    - Total Fat: 0.5g

    - Saturated Fat: 0.1g

7. **Raspberries:**

- Nutritional Information (per cup):

    - Calories: 64

    - Carbohydrates: 15g

    - Dietary Fiber: 8g

    - Total Fat: 0.8g

    - Saturated Fat: 0.1g

8. **Peaches:**

- Nutritional Information (per medium-sized):

    - Calories: 58

    - Carbohydrates: 14g

    - Dietary Fiber: 2g

    - Total Fat: 0.4g

    - Saturated Fat: 0.1g

9. **Oranges:**

- Nutritional Information (per medium-sized):

  - Calories: 62

  - Carbohydrates: 15g

  - Dietary Fiber: 3g

  - Total Fat: 0.2g

  - Saturated Fat: 0g

10. **Blueberries:**

- Nutritional Information (per cup):

  - Calories: 84

  - Carbohydrates: 21g

  - Dietary Fiber: 4g

  - Total Fat: 0.5g

  - Saturated Fat: 0.1g

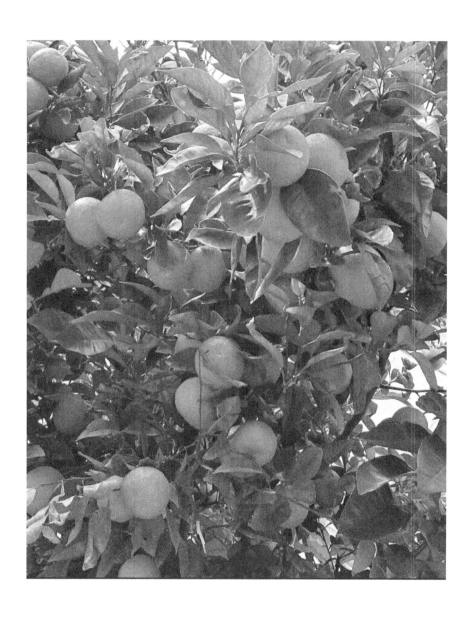

CHAPTER 6

VEGETABLES

1. **Cucumbers:**

   - Nutritional Information (per cup, sliced):

     - Calories: 16

     - Carbohydrates: 4g

     - Dietary Fiber: 1g

     - Total Fat: 0.2g

     - Saturated Fat: 0g

2. **Broccoli:**

   - Nutritional Information (per cup, chopped):

     - Calories: 55

     - Carbohydrates: 11g

     - Dietary Fiber: 5g

     - Total Fat: 0.6g

     - Saturated Fat: 0.1g

3. **Spinach:**

- Nutritional Information (per cup):

    - Calories: 7

    - Carbohydrates: 1g

    - Dietary Fiber: 1g

    - Total Fat: 0.1g

    - Saturated Fat: 0g

4. **Bell Peppers (Red or Green):**

- Nutritional Information (per cup, sliced):

    - Calories: 29

    - Carbohydrates: 7g

    - Dietary Fiber: 3g

    - Total Fat: 0.3g

    - Saturated Fat: 0.1g

5. **Zucchini:**

- Nutritional Information (per cup, sliced):

  - Calories: 20

  - Carbohydrates: 4g

  - Dietary Fiber: 1g

  - Total Fat: 0.2g

  - Saturated Fat: 0.1g

6. **Asparagus:**

- Nutritional Information (per cup):

  - Calories: 27

  - Carbohydrates: 5g

  - Dietary Fiber: 3g

  - Total Fat: 0.2g

  - Saturated Fat: 0g

7. **Tomatoes:**

- Nutritional Information (per medium-sized):

    - Calories: 22

    - Carbohydrates: 5g

    - Dietary Fiber: 2g

    - Total Fat: 0.2g

    - Saturated Fat: 0g

8. **Cauliflower:**

- Nutritional Information (per cup, chopped):

    - Calories: 27

    - Carbohydrates: 6g

    - Dietary Fiber: 3g

    - Total Fat: 0.3g

    - Saturated Fat: 0.1g

9. **Carrots:**

- Nutritional Information (per medium-sized):

    - Calories: 25

    - Carbohydrates: 6g

    - Dietary Fiber: 2g

    - Total Fat: 0.2g

    - Saturated Fat: 0g

10. **Kale:**

- Nutritional Information (per cup, chopped):

    - Calories: 33

    - Carbohydrates: 6g

    - Dietary Fiber: 1g

    - Total Fat: 0.5g

    - Saturated Fat: 0.1g

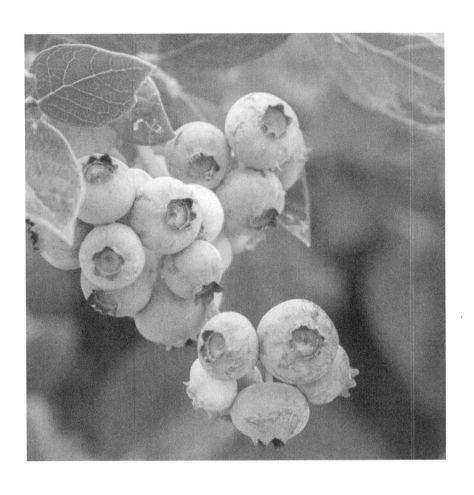

CHAPTER 7

DAIRY AND ALTERNATIVES

1. **Skim Milk:**

   - Nutritional Information (per cup):

     - Calories: 83

     - Protein: 8g

     - Carbohydrates: 12g

     - Total Fat: 0.2g

     - Saturated Fat: 0.1g

2. **Fat-Free Greek Yogurt:**

   - Nutritional Information (per 6 ounces):

     - Calories: 100

     - Protein: 15g

     - Carbohydrates: 9g

     - Total Fat: 0g

     - Saturated Fat: 0g

3. **Low-Fat Cottage Cheese:**

- Nutritional Information (per 1 cup):

    - Calories: 220

    - Protein: 28g

    - Carbohydrates: 10g

    - Total Fat: 4g

    - Saturated Fat: 2.5g

4. **Fat-Free Plain Yogurt:**

- Nutritional Information (per 6 ounces):

    - Calories: 100

    - Protein: 10g

    - Carbohydrates: 15g

    - Total Fat: 0g

    - Saturated Fat: 0g

5. **Almond Milk (Unsweetened):**

- Nutritional Information (per cup):

    - Calories: 13

    - Protein: 1g

    - Carbohydrates: 1g

    - Total Fat: 1g

    - Saturated Fat: 0g

6. **Low-Fat Ricotta Cheese:**

- Nutritional Information (per 1/2 cup):

    - Calories: 170

    - Protein: 14g

    - Carbohydrates: 6g

    - Total Fat: 10g

    - Saturated Fat: 6g

7. **Soy Milk (Unsweetened):**

- Nutritional Information (per cup):

    - Calories: 80

    - Protein: 7g

    - Carbohydrates: 4g

    - Total Fat: 4g

    - Saturated Fat: 0.5g

8. **Fat-Free Ricotta Cheese:**

- Nutritional Information (per 1/2 cup):

    - Calories: 140

    - Protein: 14g

    - Carbohydrates: 21g

    - Total Fat: 0g

    - Saturated Fat: 0g

9. **Fat-Free Cheddar Cheese:**

- Nutritional Information (per 1 ounce):

    - Calories: 45

    - Protein: 9g

    - Carbohydrates: 1g

    - Total Fat: 0g

    - Saturated Fat: 0g

10. **Low-Fat Soy Yogurt:**

- Nutritional Information (per 6 ounces):

    - Calories: 80

    - Protein: 6g

    - Carbohydrates: 14g

    - Total Fat: 1.5g

    - Saturated Fat: 0g

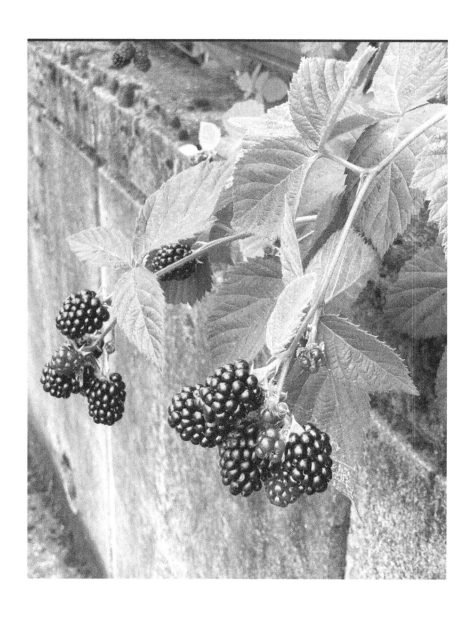

CHAPTER 8

HIGH FAT FOODS

1. **Avocado:**

   - Nutritional Information (per medium-sized avocado):

     - Calories: 234

     - Total Fat: 21g

     - Saturated Fat: 3g

     - Monounsaturated Fat: 15g

     - Polyunsaturated Fat: 2.7g

2. **Salmon (Fatty Fish):**

   - Nutritional Information (per 3.5 ounces, cooked):

     - Calories: 206

     - Total Fat: 13g

     - Saturated Fat: 3g

     - Monounsaturated Fat: 4.5g

     - Polyunsaturated Fat: 3g

3. **Cheese (Cheddar):**

- Nutritional Information (per 1 ounce):

    - Calories: 110

    - Total Fat: 9g

    - Saturated Fat: 6g

    - Monounsaturated Fat: 2.5g

    - Polyunsaturated Fat: 0.3g

4. **Walnuts:**

- Nutritional Information (per 1 ounce):

    - Calories: 185

    - Total Fat: 18g

    - Saturated Fat: 1.7g

    - Monounsaturated Fat: 2.5g

    - Polyunsaturated Fat: 13g

5. **Dark Chocolate (70-85% cocoa):**

- Nutritional Information (per 1 ounce):

  - Calories: 170

  - Total Fat: 12g

  - Saturated Fat: 7g

  - Monounsaturated Fat: 3g

  - Polyunsaturated Fat: 0.5g

6. **Pecans:**

- Nutritional Information (per 1 ounce):

  - Calories: 196

  - Total Fat: 20g

  - Saturated Fat: 1.8g

  - Monounsaturated Fat: 11g

  - Polyunsaturated Fat: 6g

7. **Full-Fat Greek Yogurt:**

- Nutritional Information (per 7 ounces):

  - Calories: 190

  - Total Fat: 10g

  - Saturated Fat: 7g

  - Monounsaturated Fat: 2.6g

  - Polyunsaturated Fat: 0.3g

8. **Macadamia Nuts:**

- Nutritional Information (per 1 ounce):

  - Calories: 204

  - Total Fat: 23g

  - Saturated Fat: 3.5g

  - Monounsaturated Fat: 16g

  - Polyunsaturated Fat: 0.5g

9. **Olive Oil:**

- Nutritional Information (per tablespoon):

    - Calories: 120

    - Total Fat: 14g

    - Saturated Fat: 2g

    - Monounsaturated Fat: 10g

    - Polyunsaturated Fat: 1.5g

10. **Coconut Oil:**

- Nutritional Information (per tablespoon):

    - Calories: 120

    - Total Fat: 14g

    - Saturated Fat: 12g

    - Monounsaturated Fat: 1g

    - Polyunsaturated Fat: 0.2g

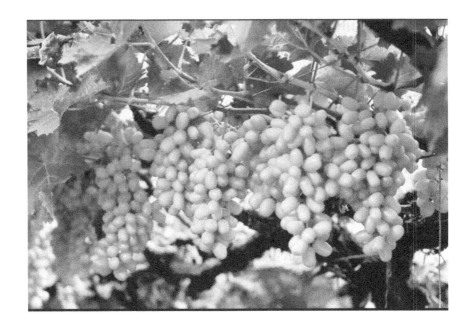

CONCLUSION

As our culinary journey through the world of Low-Fat living reaches its conclusion, I find myself overwhelmed with gratitude for the opportunity to share these recipes and insights with you. This isn't just the end of a book; it's a stepping stone towards a healthier, more vibrant you. The aromas that have danced through these pages, the flavors that have come alive in your kitchen, and the nourishment that has seeped into your body—all of these are the echoes of a transformative experience.

As we bid adieu to these pages, I want to leave you with a heartfelt reminder. Your decision to embrace Low Fat living isn't just about dieting; it's a commitment to a lifestyle that prioritizes your well-being. It's a promise to yourself—that you deserve to feel light, energetic, and joyful every single day.

But our journey doesn't end here; it's merely a transition to the next chapter of your culinary adventure. I am eager to hear about your experiences, the flavors you relished, and the changes you've noticed in your body and spirit. Your feedback is not just welcomed; it's cherished. Share your thoughts, your challenges, and your triumphs. Let this be a conversation, a community bound by the common pursuit of a healthier, more fulfilling life.

Remember, the kitchen is your canvas, and each recipe is an opportunity to create a masterpiece of well-being. The power to transform your life is in your hands, in the choices you make every day. Let the journey continue, let the flavors linger, and let the nourishment be a constant companion on your path to vitality.

Thank you for allowing me to be a part of your wellness journey. May your days be filled with the vibrant energy that stems from wholesome living, and may your kitchen forever be a sanctuary of health and joy.

BONUS CHAPTER 1

HEALTHY LOW-FAT RECIPE

Grilled Lemon Herb Chicken

- **Cooking Time:** 20 minutes

- **Servings:** 4

Ingredients:

- 4 boneless, skinless chicken breasts

- 2 tablespoons fresh lemon juice

- 1 tablespoon olive oil

- 2 cloves garlic, minced

- 1 teaspoon dried thyme

- Salt and pepper to taste

Instructions:

1. Preheat the grill to medium-high heat.

2. In a bowl, mix lemon juice, olive oil, garlic, thyme, salt, and pepper.

3. Coat chicken breasts with the marinade.

4. Grill chicken for about 8-10 minutes per side or until cooked through.

5. Serve hot.

Nutritional Information: Calories: 180, Protein: 25g, Carbohydrates: 2g, Total Fat: 8g, Saturated Fat: 1.5g

Quinoa and Black Bean Salad

- **Cooking Time:** 25 minutes

- **Servings:** 6

Ingredients:

- 1 cup quinoa, cooked

- 1 can (15 oz) black beans, drained and rinsed

- 1 cup cherry tomatoes, halved

- 1 cucumber, diced

- 1/4 cup red onion, finely chopped

- 2 tablespoons fresh lime juice

- 1 tablespoon olive oil

Instructions:

1. In a large bowl, combine quinoa, black beans, tomatoes, cucumber, and red onion.

2. In a small bowl, whisk together lime juice, olive oil, salt, and pepper.

3. Pour dressing over the salad and toss gently.

4. Chill before serving.

Nutritional Information: Calories: 180, Protein: 7g, Carbohydrates: 30g, Total Fat: 5g, Saturated Fat: 0.7g

Baked Lemon Garlic Tilapia

- **Cooking Time:** 15 minutes
- **Servings:** 2

Ingredients:

- 2 tilapia fillets
- 2 tablespoons fresh lemon juice
- 1 tablespoon olive oil
- 2 cloves garlic, minced
- 1 teaspoon dried oregano

Instructions:

1. Preheat the oven to 400°F (200°C).
2. Place tilapia fillets on a baking sheet.
3. In a small bowl, mix lemon juice, olive oil, garlic, oregano, salt, and pepper.
4. Brush the mixture over tilapia.
5. Bake for 12-15 minutes or until fish flakes easily.

Nutritional Information: Calories: 150, Protein: 25g, Carbohydrates: 1g, Total Fat: 5g, Saturated Fat: 0.8g

Vegetable Stir-Fry with Brown Rice

- **Cooking Time:** 20 minutes

- **Servings:** 4

Ingredients:

- 2 cups mixed vegetables (broccoli, bell peppers, carrots)

- 1 tablespoon low-sodium soy sauce

- 1 tablespoon olive oil

- 1 teaspoon fresh ginger, minced

- 2 cloves garlic, minced

- 2 cups cooked brown rice

Instructions:

1. Heat olive oil in a wok or skillet over medium-high heat.

2. Add ginger and garlic, sauté for 1 minute.

3. Add mixed vegetables and stir-fry until tender-crisp.

4. Stir in soy sauce and cook for an additional 2 minutes.

5. Serve over cooked brown rice.

Nutritional Information: Calories: 180, Protein: 5g, Carbohydrates: 35g, Total Fat: 4g, Saturated Fat: 0.5g

Turkey and Veggie Stuffed Peppers

- **Cooking Time:** 40 minutes
- **Servings:** 6

Ingredients:

- 6 bell peppers, halved and seeds removed
- 1 lb lean ground turkey
- 1 cup quinoa, cooked
- 1 cup black beans, drained and rinsed
- 1 cup corn kernels
- 1 cup salsa
- 1 teaspoon cumin

Instructions:

1. Preheat the oven to 375°F (190°C).
2. In a skillet, cook ground turkey until browned.
3. In a large bowl, combine turkey, cooked quinoa, black beans, corn, salsa, cumin, salt, and pepper.
4. Stuff each pepper half with the mixture.
5. Bake for 25-30 minutes or until peppers are tender.

Nutritional Information: Calories: 240, Protein: 20g, Carbohydrates: 30g, Total Fat: 5g, Saturated Fat: 1g

Chickpea and Spinach Curry

- **Cooking Time:** 25 minutes

- **Servings:** 4

Ingredients:

- 1 can (15 oz) chickpeas, drained and rinsed
- 2 cups fresh spinach
- 1 onion, finely chopped
- 2 tomatoes, diced
- 1 tablespoon curry powder
- 1 teaspoon cumin
- 1 teaspoon turmeric
- 1 teaspoon ginger, minced
- 1 can (14 oz) light coconut milk

Instructions:

1. In a large skillet, sauté onion until translucent.
2. Add curry powder, cumin, turmeric, and ginger; cook for 1 minute.
3. Stir in chickpeas, tomatoes, and coconut milk.
4. Simmer for 15 minutes, then add spinach and cook until wilted.

Nutritional Information: Calories: 220, Protein: 9g, Carbohydrates: 28g, Total Fat: 8g, Saturated Fat: 4g

Low-Fat Chicken and Vegetable Stir-Fry

- **Cooking Time:** 25 minutes

- **Servings:** 4

Ingredients:

- 1 lb boneless, skinless chicken breast, sliced

- 2 cups broccoli florets

- 1 red bell pepper, sliced

- 1 carrot, julienned

- 1 tablespoon low-sodium soy sauce

- 1 tablespoon hoisin sauce

- 1 tablespoon cornstarch

- 1 teaspoon sesame oil

- 2 cloves garlic, minced

Instructions:

1. In a bowl, mix soy sauce, hoisin sauce, cornstarch, and sesame oil.

2. Heat a wok or skillet over high heat; stir-fry chicken until cooked.

3. Add garlic, broccoli, bell pepper, and carrot; stir-fry for 3-4 minutes.

4. Pour the sauce over the stir-fry and cook for an additional 2 minutes.

Nutritional Information: Calories: 240, Protein: 30g, Carbohydrates: 15g, Total Fat: 7g, Saturated Fat: 1g

Lentil and Vegetable Soup

- **Cooking Time:** 30 minutes
- **Servings:** 6

Ingredients:

- 1 cup dry lentils, rinsed
- 1 onion, chopped
- 2 carrots, diced
- 2 celery stalks, chopped
- 3 cloves garlic, minced
- 1 can (14 oz) diced tomatoes
- 6 cups vegetable broth
- 1 teaspoon cumin
- 1 teaspoon smoked paprika
- Salt and pepper to taste

Instructions:

1. In a large pot, sauté onion, carrots, celery, and garlic until softened.

2. Add lentils, tomatoes, vegetable broth, cumin, smoked paprika, salt, and pepper.

3. Bring to a boil, then reduce heat and simmer for 20-25 minutes.

Nutritional Information: Calories: 220, Protein: 13g, Carbohydrates: 39g, Total Fat: 1g, Saturated Fat: 0g

Shrimp and Vegetable Stir-Fry

- **Cooking Time:** 20 minutes

- **Servings:** 4

Ingredients:

- 1 lb shrimp, peeled and deveined

- 2 cups broccoli florets

- 1 bell pepper, sliced

- 1 zucchini, sliced

- 2 tablespoons low-sodium soy sauce

- 1 tablespoon hoisin sauce

- 1 tablespoon olive oil

- 1 teaspoon ginger, minced

- 2 cloves garlic, minced

Instructions:

1. Heat olive oil in a wok or skillet over medium-high heat.

2. Add shrimp and cook until pink; remove from the pan.

3. In the same pan, stir-fry broccoli, bell pepper, zucchini, ginger, and garlic.

4. Add cooked shrimp back to the pan, then stir in soy sauce and hoisin sauce.

Nutritional Information: Calories: 180, Protein: 22g, Carbohydrates: 10g, Total Fat: 6g, Saturated Fat: 1g

Roasted Vegetable Medley

- **Cooking Time:** 30 minutes

- **Servings:** 4

Ingredients:

- 2 cups baby potatoes, halved

- 1 cup baby carrots

- 1 cup cherry tomatoes

- 1 zucchini, sliced

- 1 yellow squash, sliced

- 2 tablespoons olive oil

- 1 teaspoon dried thyme

- 1 teaspoon garlic powder

- Salt and pepper to taste

Instructions:

1. Preheat the oven to 400°F (200°C).

2. In a large bowl, toss potatoes, carrots, tomatoes, zucchini, and yellow squash with olive oil, thyme, garlic powder, salt, and pepper.

3. Spread the vegetables on a baking sheet.

4. Roast for 25-30 minutes or until vegetables are golden and tender.

Nutritional Information: Calories: 160, Protein: 3g, Carbohydrates: 22g, Total Fat: 7g, Saturated Fat: 1g

IF YOU WANT MORE RECIPES, YOU CAN CHECK OUT

OTHER BOOKS BY THE AUTHOR

LOW SODIUM COOKBOOK FOR SENIORS

LOW SODIUM SLOW COOKER COOKBOOK

RENAL DIET AIR FRYER COOKBOOK FOR SENIORS

DIABETIC RENAL DIET COOKBOOK FOR NEWLY

DAIGNOSED

TO GET ACCESS TO MORE BOOKS BY THE AUTHOR

SCAN THE QR CODE

BONUS CHAPTER 2

21-DAY MEAL PLAN

Day	Breakfast	Lunch	Dinner	Snack
1	Greek Yogurt Parfait	Grilled Chicken Salad	Baked Lemon Herb Tilapia	Apple slices with Almond Butter
2	Oatmeal with Berries	Quinoa and Black Bean Salad	Turkey and Veggie Stuffed Peppers	Carrot Sticks with Hummus
3	Scrambled Egg Whites	Lentil and Vegetable Soup	Shrimp and Vegetable Stir-Fry	Greek Yogurt with Berries
4	Whole Grain Toast with Avocado	Chickpea and Spinach Curry	Baked Lemon Garlic Chicken	Mixed Nuts

5	Smoothie with Spinach, Banana, and Low-Fat Yogurt	Brown Rice and Vegetable Stir-Fry	Roasted Vegetable Medley	Cottage Cheese with Pineapple
6	Low-Fat Greek Yogurt with Granola	Grilled Salmon with Asparagus	Vegetable and Tofu Stir-Fry	Orange Slices
7	Whole Wheat Pancakes with Berries	Quinoa Salad with Chickpeas	Turkey and Vegetable Skewers	Celery Sticks with Peanut Butter
8	Egg White Veggie Omelette	Lentil and Brown Rice Bowl	Baked Cod with Lemon	Cherry Tomatoes with Mozzarella
9	Cottage Cheese with Fruit	Chicken and Vegetable Wrap	Broccoli and Mushroom Stir-Fry	Banana with Almond Butter

10	Overnight Oats with Chia Seeds	Zucchini Noodles with Pesto	Grilled Chicken with Quinoa	Cucumber Slices with Yogurt Dip
11	Smoothie with Mango, Banana, and Low-Fat Yogurt	Black Bean and Vegetable Quesadilla	Baked Tilapia with Herbs	Apple slices with Cottage Cheese
12	Low-Fat Yogurt with Berries	Chickpea Salad	Turkey and Quinoa Stuffed Bell Peppers	Carrot and Cucumber Sticks with Hummus
13	Whole Grain Toast with Peanut Butter	Grilled Veggie Wrap	Lentil and Vegetable Curry	Mixed Berries
14	Egg White Scramble	Brown Rice Bowl	Baked Chicken Breast	Greek Yogurt Parfait

	with Spinach	with Stir-Fried Tofu		with Granola
15	Oat Bran Porridge with Almond Milk	Shrimp and Vegetable Stir-Fry	Quinoa and Black Bean Bowl	Celery Sticks with Cream Cheese
16	Cottage Cheese with Pineapple	Mixed Greens Salad with Grilled Chicken	Roasted Vegetable Medley	Apple Slices with Peanut Butter
17	Smoothie with Berries, Spinach, and Low-Fat Yogurt	Turkey and Vegetable Stir-Fry	Baked Lemon Herb Cod	Greek Yogurt with Almond Butter
18	Avocado Toast on Whole Wheat Bread	Lentil Soup	Grilled Salmon with Lemon	Carrot and Cucumber Sticks with Hummus

19	Scrambled Egg Whites with Tomatoes	Quinoa Salad with Chickpeas	Vegetable and Tofu Stir-Fry	Orange Slices with Almonds
20	Whole Wheat Pancakes with Blueberries	Turkey and Quinoa Stuffed Bell Peppers	Baked Chicken with Asparagus	Cottage Cheese with Mixed Berries
21	Greek Yogurt Parfait with Granola	Brown Rice and Vegetable Stir-Fry	Shrimp and Broccoli Stir-Fry	Celery Sticks with Yogurt Dip

Made in the USA
Las Vegas, NV
26 November 2024

12735628R00046